SEX SURVIVAL GUIDE FOR GUIDE FOR MILLENNIAL MEN

By Tala V. James

Hi there, Millennial Men!

If you're here, then you've got questions. And you'll be happy to know, I've got answers. Answers from a woman who's been with older men, men my own age and, definitely, some of you millennials. Unfortunately, it wasn't until I dated younger men that I realized what an effect social media and ever-ready porn has done to sex--and more specifically, lovemaking.

In this book you will find a quick guide to not only having amazing sex, but also the art of lovemaking and how to build those intimate bonds with the opposite sex.

Let's get started...

Chapter 1--Dating

You may think it's kind of funny that I would start with a chapter on dating--since there's an app for that. But what happens after the texting and messaging and you have to actually go and meet her face-to-face?? Nerve wracking for sure!

But you don't need to be scared about transitioning from anonymity to "date material", because I'm going to give you the basic tips you need to make sure that you put your best qualities forward, and ways to know if there's a "spark" or not.

First, we're going to talk about what you wear and what you decide to do for a first date (after the first date this all comes a little easier, but the first date is always the worst).

Before you can go on that date, you have to ask her out first. Of course, you can do this by text, messaging, or verbally--it really doesn't matter which way you decide to do it. But when you decide to ask a girl out, you need to make it as non-stalkerish as possible.

You may have been watching this girl for months in your English 101 class or you may work with her or you may have been friends for years, either way, you don't want to come off like you've been researching her. This will give you a high "creep rating" and will sink you before you get a chance.

I realize it's hard to not go overboard when she's been on your radar a lot longer than you've been on hers, but you MUST not let her know that you have been secretly pining over her. You can tell her that you think she's pretty (not gorgeous--that's too much at first!), that you like her smile, or that you admire the short story that she presented in class--these are all safe ways to let her know that you like her and maybe want to get to know her better.

Just so we're clear, other no-no's are: whistling at her, making rude remarks about her body/body parts, making other rude noises, making fun of her in front of others, pestering her, becoming obsessed with her, or touching her anywhere but her arm or her shoulder (touching at this stage should be kept to a minimum anyway).

Alternatively, things you can do to let her know you're interested: slip her a note asking her out for a drink of her choice (it's okay to offer alternatives to alcohol too--coffee, juice, etc.), ask about studying in the library with her, invite her to a group event/gathering, just talk to her for a few minutes every so often before or after class, work, etc.--the main thing here is to not go overboard with the attention and to watch for her to show interest in you.

And please don't take it personally if she doesn't seem interested!! She may already be dating someone else, may be gay, may have other stressful things going on in her life at the moment, OR she may just not feel a spark--and a spark isn't something that you can force. We all must realize that we are not going to click with everyone, in actuality, we aren't going to click with MOST people--so don't let it get to you if she doesn't seem interested.

If you have tried a couple of times to get her attention or to see if she's interested and you just aren't sure, it is certainly acceptable for you to very clearly (but quietly) ask if she would consider going out on a date. If she says "yes", then great! But if she says "no", then you should be gracious about it and not bug her about it any longer. You can still be social with her in groups, but don't single her out.

Once you ask a girl if she'd like to go out on a date, she will remember it, and if, in the future, she becomes interested or free to date, then she will still be aware that you like her, and she can hit you up for the date this time.

One final tactic that I want to mention that works some of the time, and is very useful for those guys who are shy or don't take rejection well, is to use a mutual friend to be the go-between. It's very effective in two ways: your friend will be able to answer some of the questions that the girl may have about what kind of person you are; and your friend will possibly be able to explain a little more about why she refuses a date or can give you tips on her likes/dislikes if she agrees.

Now, after she's accepted that initial "coffee" date, the next thing to worry about is how to dress.

This should be a no-brainer...wear whatever you're comfortable in that fits the level of fanciness of the establishment you're going to AND make sure everything you're wearing is clean and doesn't smell or have stains on it (this includes underarm sweat stains). You don't have to put a lot of money into your wardrobe, but you need to have clean, fresh smelling clothes since women can be turned off by certain smells. This by no means gives you the chance to bathe in cologne!! No, no, no! Cologne should be used sparingly, and soap and toothpaste used copiously!

And that's about it on this issue.

Next, where are you going to go and what are you going to do? This doesn't have to be decided before you actually meet up, but if things go well with coffee then you might want to have another activity kind of figured out to suggest at the end of the coffee.

Usually this possible "after coffee" activity should be something that lasts about an hour, but definitely no more than two hours. Only ask about doing something after coffee if you're getting clear signals that she's interested AND only if it seems appropriate. For instance, if she should say that she has an exam that she has to study for or she has work early in the morning, then you shouldn't be suggesting an extended first date. Be respectful of her schedule and just ask at the end of the date if it would be okay to get her number or message her on social media. If she seems a little reluctant, or you're not sure you can read her signals, it is certainly acceptable to give her your number so she can decide later if she'd like to get in touch again.

The number one thing you can do at this point is play a little hard to get, or at least not be **too** overly eager. Letting her feel comfortable with you is the first step in building a dating relationship. PLUS, as I'll explain later, the anticipation will enhance things later on between the two of you if you do end up starting a relationship--stay tuned to find out why!

Next thing we need to talk about is your ability to keep track of her on social media without her knowing it, and how this should be a no-no if you want to have a shot at a real relationship with her.

Successful couples lead their own lives and choose to share their life experiences with someone else--that's dating/a relationship. This will also give you both more things to talk about when you're together, so don't sabotage yourself by knowing everything there is to know about a girl in whom you're interested.

So, when do you call/text/message her to see about another date if you didn't already decide on it at the coffee date? You need to wait at least two days--any earlier than this needs to be left up to her to initiate. If she's interested then she will get back to you within these two days, if she's not sure or maybe having some other relationship issues, then she may not get back to you. It is certainly acceptable after two days to contact her and casually ask her if she would be interested in a regular dinner date. And again, don't take it personally if she says "no".

If you make plans with her to go on a regular date, the only piece of advice I can give you on this is to split up the decision making--one of you pick the place to eat and the other pick the activity. Both of you need to try and be up for whatever the other one picks as this will give you a chance to get to know a little bit about her and she will get to know a little about you too by what each of you choose. If she picks an Italian restaurant then you can deduce that she likes that type of food. If you pick hiking as an activity then she can see that you like to do outdoor things--the rule of thumb here is don't do things that you don't like to do. Be genuine.

So, is there a time when you absolutely SHOULD speak up? Yes. The only time you need to speak up is if you have a religious reason or a medical reason for not being able to do something the other person has suggested--but you still need to be nice about it when you tell them this. If it's a religious reason you need to make sure that you don't sound judgmental. If it's a medical reason, don't go into too much detail about it at this point.

   And PLEASE, PLEASE, PLEASE do NOT post things about dating on social media until you have both decided that you're going to pursue the relationship. This is usually evident/decided around date #4--it takes that many dates to really decide if this is something to continue on to the next level, which is "steady dating". Posting things too early can actually look weird, not only to the person you're trying to date, but also everyone else you know.

That's about it on this section, now on to the nitty-gritty of sex…

Now what you've been waiting for...SEX...well, I guess not exactly **YET**, anyway.

Let me start by saying that sex on the first date should never be expected. And if your first "date" is actually a group-thing and there's drinking or drugs involved, I would steer clear of trying ANYTHING on that first date, even if she's the one trying to initiate sex. Even if you're out on a one-on-one date, or you may even be a date or two into this new relationship, the introduction of anything that could alter her decision-making abilities should be a reason to NOT pursue sex on that date.

If you want to actually pursue any type of relationship with a girl, you need to make sure that you protect her from possible poor decisions made when she's under the influence, instead of taking advantage of the situation. She will think much more highly of you if you keep her safe and treat her well than if she wakes up next to you regretting the whole night.

Once you and she have begun having sex in your relationship on a regular basis, then it is acceptable to have sex after a night out drinking or using drugs. But even then, you should make sure that she's still coherent enough to give consent. How do you know if she's still with it enough to do it? Ask her questions that she should still be able to do even if she's a little inebriated (do not use yes and no questions). Examples: simple math (25+25+30?), spelling (spell "mathematics"), or ask her to read you the label on something (if this takes too long or she's unable to sound things out then it should be a no-go).

Here's the added plus when she's coherent enough to consent...she will be able to be an **active** participant AND she will remember it. Sex is so much hotter when both people can do their part! And how great is it going to be for your ego the next morning if she doesn't even remember it? In addition, if you have to try and explain it all to her the next morning, this could be embarrassing for both of you and actually drive a wedge between you if she feels she can't trust you because of it.

Here's the nitty-gritty that I promised:

I cannot emphasize this enough fellas...by making **her** feel good, **your** sex life will be a hundred times better!

I'm going to go against popular "pop culture" beliefs right now, but I just have to--because what you believe right now about how your sex life should look like is probably all wrong. It's not exactly your fault...it's more about what you've been conditioned into thinking that sex should look like by watching only ridiculous, male-filmed porn.

The majority of the porn that you see on the web is directed by men, filmed by men, and written by men--and many of these men are sick puppies! Their films are made to show the most ridiculous things they can think up. The porn industry generally portrays women in a way that leads men to think that women are just there to be used and that they get enjoyment out of this--NOT TRUE.

Women do not get any enjoyment out of the majority of the crazy positions and angles that you see, they definitely don't get turned on by blowjobs, and they cannot tolerate sex for super long periods of time. These are FACTS, so heed them.

You also need to take the pressure off yourself.

There's no need to have an extensive repertoire of moves, positions, or dirty talk to satisfy a woman. In fact, if you have two or three moves and/or positions that turn us on, we're good with that. As for dirty talk...well that depends on the woman. If you want to know what to say to her while lovemaking, take your cues from her. And, just so you know, most men average about seven minutes for actual penetration--and THIS is just fine with women as long as there's been enough foreplay.

Let's break some of these things down a little further. We'll tackle the **sexy talk** first.

Basically, all you have to do is listen to what SHE says during sex and try to give her about the same level of raunchiness and frequency. Is it sexy talk or graphic talk? It's also important to pay attention to her tone of voice. Does she have a louder, more aggressive way of talking or is it more whispered in your ear when your heads are close together?

Does this mean that if you're really turned on by certain words, or by words being said a certain way, that you just have to forget about what you want? No, but you want to take care that you don't go so far away from what SHE likes that it's a turnoff for her.

Then, over time, you can begin to ask her how she feels about different things, including the way you talk to each other during sex. If you really like to have raunchy talk then you can just ask her if she'd be up to it as a roleplaying bit. She might agree, and she might not. But it's definitely something you can bring up from time to time and keep talking about as your relationship progresses.

Now we're going to talk about the **pre-sex moves**.

The first moves you're going to use are actually moves that you need to be using all evening BEFORE any clothes come off. The basic moves that will make a woman feel special and also get her in a romantic mood are: holding hands, your arm loosely around her shoulder when sitting next to each other, running your hand on her thigh (do not go any higher than mid-thigh), letting her put her feet in your lap, etc. Keep in mind that you don't have to constantly be touching her, but doing these little things occasionally, and when it seems natural and relaxing to do so, can help her make a deeper connection with you.

Making a deeper connection is necessary for women when deciding to continue to date someone, but too much can make her feel smothered and is a real turn-off. So, you definitely don't want to pressure her into any of this--that means you'll have to be keeping a watchful eye on her body language. If she pulls away or stiffens up, then you might want to back off a bit and give her more time and/or space. Meaningful eye contact and sexy, slightly teasing smiles are also important--just make sure you don't use these constantly or you'll make her uncomfortable; it'll seem like you're staring, and a constant smile is just...well...goofy.

It may seem silly that these things make a difference, but you have to remember that biologically it takes women's bodies a lot longer than men's to warm up to having sex. Why not do a few loving gestures throughout the day/night to get her body and mind on the right track and, hopefully as an added benefit for you, it will cut down on the length of time needed for foreplay later.

The next moves you're going to use come under the term "petting". I'm surprised how many millennial men have no idea how to do this! This is very important because it adds two very important elements: suspense and frustration.

You may not think that these two elements can help, but they are the things that are missing the most in our ever-ready-porn-watching-young-people. Going right into sex without any of the buildup is not near as exciting for EITHER person. The longer you can stay in this stage of anticipation, the hungrier you will both be to consummate it. (FYI: there's a ton of literature about this out there--you can learn more by reading on kama sutra.)

Here's some petting moves you can use (listed in order from start to finish):
1. barely rubbing or tickling her breasts through her shirt,
2. laying your hand on her stomach and slowly making your way under her shirt and up to her breast,
3. rubbing and/or gently cupping her breasts with her bra still between your hand and her breast,

4. slowly advancing your hand to touch her breasts inside her bra,
5. finding her nipples and gently rubbing them until they pucker/become hard,
6. rubbing her clit through her jeans until she is panting/indicating that she wants your hands inside her pants,
7. slowly unbuttoning/unzipping pants,
8. softly laying your palm on the bottom part of her stomach before slowly advancing it down below her underwear,
9. find her clit,
10. stroke just her clit with one finger (go side to side, then forward and back, then repeat as much as wanted),
11. advance your hand enough to get one or two fingers PARTIALLY inside her and slowly go in and out while applying moderate pressure with the palm of your hand on her mound/clit area.

I would recommend that you be kissing her on her lips, ears, neck, upper chest, shoulders, and several places on her face as you do these petting moves. Make it sensual and sexy. Take time to whisper to her--tell her how beautiful she is and how much you want her.

And... that's it.

Really, this is what you want to do if you're in the car after a date, laying out in the backyard under the stars, laying on the couch, or any other time that you want to try and have sex. Will it always work to get her to have sex with you? No, not always, but your chances are much better if you've taken the time to get her warmed up. And, yes, there will be those times where you just have a "quickie", but these should be few, especially in the beginning of a relationship, and NEVER the first few times.

Now for the **undressing**!

This can be a disaster if you try and rush things--so take your time. This is something that you want to do sensually the first several times you have sex, and then later, after you're both used to each other and/or you're actually sleeping in the same bed every night, you can ditch the drawn-out undressing and only use it for special occasions or after a special date.

The easiest way to undress while maintaining some sexiness in it is to take turns undressing each other while standing. There're several ways you can go about this, but the best one I've found is where you mimic each other (i.e. you slip her shirt off over her head and she does yours, you unbutton her jeans and she does yours, etc.) while continuing to kiss and caress each other.

The next best way (also standing) is to start undressing the other person as you keep kissing each other, and then quickly transition into each person taking over their own disrobing, but still kissing throughout and pausing every so often to hug bodies together. This one can cause some unintended bumping of heads, teeth, knees, etc. because you are undressing simultaneously, so be ready to just give up the kissing when clothes below the belly button have to come off.

The last, and the hardest way to get clothes off one another, is after you're already lying down. In this case it's sometimes better to just leave some of the clothing on. If either of you have a button up shirt, just leave it on but make sure it's unbuttoned so she can run her hands over your skin and you can have access to her breasts. Both of you must keep in mind that the clothing on the lower half of your bodies will have to be dealt with in a way to allow whatever sexual position you're going to use. Leaving socks on, or a leg in a pair of pants, usually is no big deal.

After you begin sleeping together on a regular basis you will likely come to bed in some sort of pajamas/nightgown. It's up to you as a couple to decide if you want to just leave tops on and ditch the bottoms--just make sure and mix it up once in a while and get completely naked for that delicious skin-on-skin.

Chapter 3--Sex, Finally!

We've finally made it to the SEX portion of this book! And, as you will see, this is the probably the shortest of the chapters. Why? Because sex is something that changes each time you do it and with each partner you do it with.

Sex should take into consideration not only what YOU like, but also what the woman likes and/or can tolerate. There are so many different positions and moves out there, that you can pick up on any website, that I don't really need to go into any of them. But what we DO need to go over is how you use them, and how you present them to her.

Contrary to what you've been led to believe by the porn industry, women generally don't enjoy being forcefully, and relentlessly, pistoned in and out of. They get greater enjoyment from a more gentle and loving form of coupling that has brief moments of more intense passion. You can't go wrong if you use a more woman-focused approach where **your moves** are guided by the woman's responses--but this only works if you take the time to "check in" with her.

For those that are still unsure what "woman-focused sex" includes, it includes the following elements: some tantalizing teasing; some medium, slower penetration; alternating times of more forceful thrusting; and use of different angles to try and tease out that coveted g-spot stimulation. This type of sexual encounter is more fulfilling, making a woman feel a deeper connection and passion for their partner--which ultimately translates into more sex for the man. Yeah!

   (I would like to make this disclaimer here before we go any further: make sure and have condoms available anywhere that you might engage in sex for the first several months of a new relationship-- i.e. bedside, bathroom, billfold, her purse, etc. There're many reasons for this, but mostly so that you don't catch or spread anything before you decide if this is going to be a long-term relationship or not. An added bonus is that your erection will end up lasting longer, so bring on the condom!)

   Now that we've covered safety, let's talk about what's next...
   You've been loving towards her all night.
   You did the petting in the car before driving to your apartment.
   You're both undressed and you have condoms handy.
   Now what do you do?...You go **back** to the petting again!

Yes, I know. You probably feel like you're backtracking and may be thinking "why do I have to do it twice?" --but think about how she reacted to the petting the first time. YES, yes! You have to get her back to that point, which won't take long since you've already gotten her mostly there before.

So, do the petting steps again (skipping the clothes part OR doing the clothes part as you undress her). Then when it comes to moving your hand down to her clit, at the same time move your kissing and nibbling down to her breasts. Be careful to use your lips and tongue mostly, and teeth very rarely and gently.

This time round when you begin touching her clitoris, you will want to do it with a little more pressure and alternating it with dipping your fingers halfway inside her vagina. Once you have her moaning with her first orgasm, go ahead and advance your finger/fingers inside as far as possible to help tip her into that full orgasm. Make sure and leave your fingers inside for a little while after her muscles stop contracting and do not touch her clit until it becomes a little less sensitive. If you go back to touching her clitoris and she flinches, wait another twenty seconds or so and try again. In those twenty seconds go back to kissing her and/or nibbling on her ears, neck, breasts, etc.

As soon as you're able to touch her clit again, this is the time to decide if you want to continue

with foreplay or try penetration. If you want to
continue foreplay, then you will need to decide if
you are going to use your finger or mouth to build
her next orgasm.   If you decide to go with
penetration, then you need to decide if you are
going to use your fingers again to penetrate her or
if you want to go ahead with intercourse. Either
way, you don't have to use everything you know in
the first sex session, or even the second. Just
make sure you always lead up to any type of
penetration with clitoral stimulation while
simultaneously using your lips and hands on the
rest of her body. And just so we're clear on when
you should be able to engage in penile-vaginal
sex, a general rule of thumb is: if she's had at
least two orgasms then you have a green-light to
proceed however quickly to the penetration stage
as you would like.

Once you've gotten to that point where you
want to use your penis in her vagina, make sure
that she's wet enough for this, and if there's a big
difference in sizes (i.e. she's smaller than you),
then you will need to take extra care in entering
her the first several times. Lubrication is key to
preventing pain that could halt sex in a second. If
you find you need extra lubrication, you can use a
lubricant specifically for this, or keep stimulating
her until there's enough natural body fluids to
allow it.

This is NOT the time to experiment with
anything other than "vanilla" sex. You are just

starting to get to know each other. Fetishes and particular turn-ons should come out slowly, and definitely LATER. Just enjoy being with a new person, and if you can't get off without one of your fantasies, then think about it in your mind as you go ahead and have sex with the person that's in front of you. Over time you can try to incorporate enough of your fantasies (**both** yours and hers) into your sex life to satisfy your needs, but until then, you're going to have to get really good at visualization.

During the penetration part of sex, keep these things in mind:

- You want to last long enough to get her to orgasm WITH you--this is the most amazing feeling for BOTH of you--yes, **you'll** enjoy it immensely too!
- You will need to go slow at first.
- Varying your speed and depth will make it more enjoyable for both of you.
- If you find she's not orgasming, and you're getting fairly close, then completely insert your penis inside her and try to angle the tip of your penis toward her belly button as you do short thrusts. This is the general location of her g-spot and you want to try and stimulate it.
- If these short, g-spot thrusts don't do the trick, try moving your tip in small circles. You will want to do a little of both and mix it

up between the g-spot thrusts and the tip circles--but don't worry about mixing it up too quickly. Do quite a few short thrusts and then do several slow circles before going back to general thrusting for a while.

- If she needs additional stimulation it is perfectly okay to encourage her to touch herself during sex in any way that she needs to--just be careful to not come off as if you don't want to be bothered with it or ordering her to do it "herself". FYI: This usually only needs to be used if you have been having a longer sex session where she's had quite a few orgasms already OR the g-spot is illusive with penile penetration.

- Once she starts orgasming, you will need to do several long, quick, strong thrusts to get yourself orgasming before hers ends. This can take some practice so don't worry if you don't always get it timed "exactly right" each and every time. As you get to know her signs (and sounds) of pre-orgasm you'll be able to get the timing worked out.

- When both of you have completed, do NOT pull out! Pulling out immediately can leave her feeling abandoned and used. By laying there holding onto one another you are conveying a sense of fulfillment and acceptance. In addition, both your bodies will begin to automatically start separating without an assistance from either of you.

Once this process starts you are now able to go ahead and slowly pull yourself out.

- There will be the condom issue to deal with at this point also. If you don't hold onto the rim of the condom it can actually pull off, so make sure that you hold onto it as you withdraw. It's handy to have, at the very least, a tissue at bedside to discard this in.
- Once the condom has been dealt with, cuddling is very important for women...and for you as well. Whether you realize it or not, adult men do not get hugs on a regular basis, unless it's from a romantic partner. This is sad, but it's only because socially it's not as acceptable for men to do this except in certain circumstances (i.e. family, very special occasions like weddings/funerals, etc.). So, take advantage of all the feel-good hormones that are swimming through both of your bodies and hug it out.
- Here's probably the MOST important part of post-sex: let her talk. This is going to be the time she'll want to talk to you the most-- and you can blame it on those feel-good hormones. She feels connected to you now. It's the best time to build your relationship, so make a big effort to talk with her for at least five to ten minutes. I realize that this may be very hard for you since those same feel-good hormones act

differently in the male body, making you sleepy. But, seriously, give her the few minutes she needs, and you'll be rewarded time and time again.

That's pretty much it about having good, connecting sex with someone for the first time. Just remember that you can't just do these things on the first encounter and then abandon everything when you have sex again. These steps are your basics, and while you can certainly add to them, it would be detrimental to your relationship to begin chucking any of them away.

When you DO decide it's time to start adding in more moves, keep in mind that most couples generally have just a few things that work for **both** of them, one or two things that turn on **each of them** separately, and then a few things that they like **to try** from time to time. Honestly, you do NOT have to be some wildman between the sheets to make a woman feel good, or to have a good time yourself.

Seriously, if you're doubting me right now, don't. What you've been conditioned to believe about sex up to this point may be hard to overcome completely, or quickly, but I'm begging you to just give it a chance. -I promise you that you'll be pleasantly surprised how turned on you'll actually get from practicing woman-focused sex. Taking the time to really pay attention to her sounds, how her body responds and moves, and what she says, will improve your sexual prowess and prove to both of you that you have what it takes to be a great lover.

Don't stop here!--keep reading to learn some more important sexual "tidbits", and to get some guidance on how to keep your sex life alive and well over time.

This chapter is going to be a mish-mash of important things to learn about sex and the female body...and a little bit you may not know about your own body, believe it or not!

<u>Let's talk about: Just Being Friends</u>

Every man hears "I just want to be friends" many, many times during their lifetime, so don't sweat it if a girl says it to you. For women there has to be this "spark". This spark is hard to explain, but it's definitely an **automatic** connection that can't be fabricated with a little bit of sexual attraction thrown in. Two people can be sexually attracted to each other, but it will soon fizzle because there's no real connection to sustain it. On the other hand, two people can have a real connection **without** the sexual attraction and these situations will retain some potential for developing into a romantic relationship. See, you can have the connection without the sexual attraction and, as two people become emotionally closer, the sexual attraction may develop later because the connection is so strong. Sooo...if she says that she just wants to be friends, don't count it out forever, and, worst-case scenario? You could end up good friends--which isn't so bad!

<u>Let's talk about: Being Friends w/Benefits</u>

This kind of relationship is a fairly new phenomenon and completely bogus on both people's part--both are just using the other until something better comes along. The guy may think this kind of arrangement is perfect, but it's really not--it can chip away at your motivation to go out there and find someone that's better for you in **all ways**. And, unbeknownst to you, it's not the same way for a woman in the same situation. Many women just don't want to be alone, or they yearn to have sex with a guy just to prove to themselves (and their girlfriends) that someone finds them attractive--but this in no way means they've quit looking for a better deal! You may also think that this type of relationship will develop into something MORE if you "just stick with it", but that's rarer than Sasquatch--so steer clear of this dead-end situation!

<u>Let's talk about: Being Good Boyfriend Material</u>

This is a hard subject as it also changes with each and every partner. Again, this is where you need to watch your girl for things that will clue you in on what she likes and doesn't like. This is also where you need to make sure that you aren't putting on such a facade that you can't keep it up. You need to be as much like yourself as possible--because you don't want to date a poser and you also don't want to be one. When you put time into a relationship you should be getting to know the REAL person, versus some fake-ass persona that will disappear with the first sign of true commitment.

So, what makes a guy a good boyfriend? Here's a list of the basics:
- Be willing to talk about things--this should be an investigative discussion, or at the very least a few questions, before giving her your opinion and then letting her voice hers (or vice versa). If a decision needs to be made, then it should be made on what makes the MOST sense. It may take several different discussions before things are better, but that's because it allows enough time for both of you to think about things that were said.
- Be willing to compromise--it is NOT about "winning"...nobody "wins" if one person in the couple is upset or angry. Disclaimer: this should not be a one-sided thing--if you need to remind her that you often compromise, and you would like her to compromise on something else then that is fine, BUT don't expect to get a compromise on things that can jeopardize your/her

safety or the safety of your relationship with her.

- Listen without judgement--if you don't know what to do to help her, just say you don't know.
- Support her in her decisions--but first a discussion (see above on talking about things).
- Be honest. Just be sure to use a little tact and steer away from being "brutally".
- Be willing to treat her well without going overboard--how you treat her every single day, day in and day out, speaks much louder than what you do a few times a year for special occasions.
- Remember important things and follow through. If she's asked you to do something AND you agree, just follow through--she's counting on you.
- Offer to help.
- Be willing to accept help.
- Be willing to help out equally at home (if you're living together and she also works).
- Reciprocate actions (i.e. if she makes a big deal about your b-day you should make one for hers, if she gives you a backrub after a particularly hard day then you should do the same for her, etc.).
- Leave her little notes, write love letters, send her texts that boost her self-esteem--

women in general need more reassurance than men that they are attractive and that you love/care about them. Doing something like this once or twice a day is enough, more than that and it becomes tiresome.

- Let her tell you secrets and keep them--it's important to have that person that you can vent to and not worry about what you say getting back to the person you said them about. She can't find this assurance with her girlfriends, no matter how good a girlfriend is, there's always that risk.

- Do little things to show her you're paying attention--this is truly about the little things! If you notice that she likes something (i.e. granola in her yogurt, a certain place on the sofa, etc.) then try to let her have those things without having to ask. Those little considerations mean so much to women (because they make those little accommodations for you all the time, usually without you realizing it).

Anytime you are unsure of what to do in a situation, always go back to talking it out. There's no way I can possibly address every single hiccup that you are going to encounter when you interact with women, but rest assured that talking to them in a civil manner will reap greater understanding no matter what the issue.

Let's talk about: Masturbation

Masturbation is something women know all men do BUT we don't want to generally be audience to it. This is something that you need to do in a way that we don't hear it or have to clean anything up afterwards. So...do it while we're out, please.

As for female masturbation, it exists...but we won't do it in front of you unless you ask, and some women feel too embarrassed to do it even then. If this is a turn on for you then you need to let her know that, but only after your relationship is well-established. You can even start it for her and have her join in, just don't push her or she'll end up worried about it instead of enjoying it.

Let's talk about: Porn

I can't say enough about porn!
In general, porn has been the downfall of sex. When men use porn videos to learn about sex, they miss out on all the most important stuff! And the porn that most men watch these days is, frankly, bullshit. Almost every scene encourages men to pound women into submission before pulling out and wasting their orgasm on a "sperm facial". Porn has also desensitized men, AND women, to what sex is supposed to really be about--a connection not only on a physical level but also on an emotional level.

Remember when we were in chemistry class, we learned that paired bonds are stronger than others? So, it should make sense that stronger bonds are built between two people when they pair up a loving emotional attachment with a satisfying sexual connection. We have loads of men out here wondering why they can't build a relationship with a woman, and women are discouraged because they're not getting any fulfillment at all from men. This is what's making dating so hard to do, and why so many people are ending up alone and wondering what's gone wrong--we've forgotten about how important it is to have a true connection with the person we're having sex with.

So, even after all of this, if you're still wanting to use porn as part of your sex life, or if you want to actually SEE what I've been talking about in this Guide, then I would recommend porn that is written, directed, and produced by women. Even though this is a fairly new genre, you can do an internet search and find "women directed porn" without any difficulty--it's just not going to be the first thing that pops up on most porn sites. And if watching porn with your girlfriend is something that you would like to do, then this is the type you'll want to watch, as it will appeal to her more than other types of porn.

All of this being said, I still cannot stress enough how important it is for BOTH of you to view porn as little as possible. Even though women-made porn is more realistic, it's still porn, and it can make you and your partner feel like you're missing something, when in reality you're not. Besides...it's so much more fun to just explore each other's body and to figure out things you want to try on your own--unscripted.

<u>Let's talk about: Fetishes/fantasies</u>

   Okay, I have to be honest with you here...fetishes and fantasies are considered two different things, and there's literally thousands of them. Since I can't possibly go over each and every one of them, or anticipate any new one you may have discovered, I'll just address them both fairly briefly here.
   So, here's the brief: fantasies are always fine as long as they are restricted to inside your head, and fetishes are...just fantasies out in the open.
   The only advice I can give you about fetishes is to make sure and save these for when you and your partner are more comfortable with each other, and start slow. Bring up one thing at a time and see what she thinks about it. Some she may want to try and then decide it's not for her, some she may try and they're keepers. Just never know. (Oh, and make sure to ask her about hers too!)

<u>Let's talk about: Anal</u>

This is one of those sex acts that has been done up so terrible in porn that many women think that it's one of two things: 1) too painful to try; 2) it's expected and it's purely for the enjoyment of the man. I see this as a true pity, because when the anus is stimulated correctly, for women AND men, it can be a great enhancement to your repertoire of moves.

Since this is something that almost every man and woman will experience at some time during sex, it's important that you have clear-cut instructions on how to make it enjoyable instead of something to cringe about.

I think that it's easiest to go at this by giving you step-by-step guidelines that you can improve upon as your skills get better with practice. The only hard rule about this is: don't do anything by force. Anytime she gasps or makes any other noise that might signify pain, stop and ask her if it's alright. If she says yes, then continue on to the next step. If she says no, then you can ask her if she wants you to stop or just continue what you were doing before it started hurting.

It's important to follow these steps **in order**:
1. Using your wet finger press lightly against her butthole without penetrating, then release. Repeat this several times (like you're pressing down on a computer key with the pad of your finger).

2. After a little time, you can try introducing your fingertip into the hole.
3. If she's agreeable, you can advance the finger.
4. At this stage you can try introducing more fingers, but this will be something you have to work up to if she doesn't have much anal experience. You can also skip this step of adding more fingers and go to #5 instead OR you can flip back and forth between this step and step #5--totally up to you and her.
5. Begin moving your finger(s) in and out, but not fast. You can gradually work up to a faster pace, but keep in mind that as soon as it begins hurting, she will more than likely tell you to stop.
6. Now you can either keep going until she orgasms as part of your foreplay OR you can be warming her up for penile anal sex. If this is part of your foreplay and you are not going to be doing anal, the perfect time to do this anal play is after you've stimulated her clitoris and vagina but before you have vaginal sex. If you're wanting to have anal, then this is the time for you to ask permission and make sure you have more lubrication than you might think is necessary. Get the lube all over your penis and a small amount on her anus as well. (Sorry, boys, but vaginal fluids and

spit aren't enough to keep it wet enough for her to let you possibly keep going for long-- trust me on this!)

7. Holding your penis, press gently up against her anus with the tip. It should slide in with little difficulty, but if she tightens up then you will have to stop until she relaxes. Some women only like a very little inside and some like a lot--again it's different for every woman, and also for every single encounter (even with the same woman).

8. Once you've made it in as far as possible then you should take a few seconds to get in a comfortable position for you to be able to begin slow thrusts. Keep in mind that if she's only let you put the tip in then you will more than likely have to keep a hand on your penis throughout so that it doesn't pull out completely.

9. After she has begun to show signs that she's enjoying this then you can begin to go a little faster. You can also try every so often to advance in a little further as her anal canal and sphincters relax, but you will want to take pause and do this slowly instead of part of your fast thrusting.

10. When it comes to ejaculating you will have to be careful to not get too enthusiastic and go too deep, too hard or too fast. Unlike vaginal sex, this takes a better level of self-control, so if you're lacking in this I would

recommend waiting until you have more of it.

11. Unlike vaginal sex, it can be painful for the woman when you pull out so make sure and let your penis get softer and hold onto the condom (if you used one) so it doesn't get lost inside her. As you back out, do so at a medium speed, too slow and too fast both hurt more. It also helps if you wait for her body to try and expel your penis, as this is a natural reflex and it helps with the exit.

A few general tidbits to remember about anal sex:

- You cannot go back and forth between her vagina/clit and her asshole--you will give her an infection. If you want to go back up to the vaginal area after playing with her backside then go wash your hands/penis.
- You might want to use a condom, as this protects you and her, but in this case it also makes clean up easier afterwards.
- You never know when you'll end up pulling a small nugget of poo out, or when your ejaculate may cause an enema-like effect-- so it's helpful to put a towel underneath her hips to catch anything.
- Some women are going to be bloated and more tender in the anal region during PMS and their period, so anal is not always

going to be an option at all times of the month. Showing her some consideration during this time of the month will have you reaping the rewards for being such a unselfish bloke!

- You can use sex toys and vibrators in and/or around the anus, just make sure that they are not too big and that you don't insert them so far that you risk losing them inside her (which is easy to do because of the lube). You will also want to start out small and go easy with the toys.

- Do not expect a woman to go "ass-to-mouth" on your penis. This is one of those stunts that you see in porn that's not always what it seems. Most times they have taken a break for the man to wash up before the woman gives him a blowjob--and you won't be able to tell due to the expertise they have with splicing it all together to look seamless. So don't ever expect this trick.

- For some reason though, some people DO like to turn their partner on by licking the other person's asshole. If this is something that your partner does for you, be a caring lover by making sure you wash it well right before you have sex. Baby wipes work well for this but can leave a weird taste, so if you're extra considerate, give it a rinse.

- Don't be surprised if a woman is the one that initiates anal play on YOU during a blowjob. Women now know that the taint and anal areas on men are full of nerve endings and they will play with them to get you more turned on. If this is not something that you're into, then just nicely tell her or use your hands to move her hands where you want them. It's okay for you to say "no" too.
- Last, but not least, using **actual** anal lube. Many people will use tons of different things as lubrication for anal sex, but these other products can actually mess both of you up--from rashes, to burning, to infections. It's just safer to use the products made specifically for this kind of sex play.

<u>Let's talk about: Blowjobs</u>

Blowjobs used to be taboo, but they became all the rage in the 1990s-2000s. Many teens engaged in them because they viewed it as "not really having sex". Sadly, all this did was bolster young men's opinion that women are useable, and disposable, after getting what they wanted. Before that time, blowjobs were only something that long-term couples did, and they only did it occasionally, usually on special occasions, believe it or not. Now blowjobs are commonplace and are actually expected. This really isn't how it should be, though.

In the porn industry men are constantly forcing women to do blowjobs, including performing the deepthroat form of this until they are gagging and crying. It's not how it is in real life and any man that tries to duplicate these rougher tactics will not have any woman sticking around.

So, lets go over the things that you should know regarding a BJ:

- Don't expect her to do this on your first sexual encounter together. You also don't have to go down on her the first time either. Heck! Neither one of you HAVE to give the other oral sex, but it IS unfair to have your partner do you and then not reciprocate. So keep this in mind if you don't want to go down on her EVER but you want her to go down on you.
- If, after a few times together, she hasn't already given you a blowjob, or at the very least kissed around on your penis, then it is acceptable for you to ask/suggest it. Some women will let you know right then if it's going to be something that they aren't willing to do, and that leaves you to decide if you're still willing to stay in it without having that as an option.
- Not all women are good at giving BJs, and those that are just starting out WILL get

better. It's certainly okay to give some little indications of what feels good, but you run the risk of her not doing it ever again if you criticize her. So how do you let her know what feels good? I'm sure she's going to get some indications just from the involuntary sounds you make during the blowjob, so don't hold back, but also don't do any fake noises--we can tell the difference. You can also use the female-made porn videos I mentioned before to help you out with getting her to try different techniques, that's if you're BOTH into watching them. Again, though, you have to watch HOW you try to get her to change her technique. For instance, you can say "Oooh, I'd like you to try that sometime", but it wouldn't be good to say "That looks like that'd feel better than what you did the other night"--totally different tones. Always strive to be gentle with your words when talking about sex.

- It's sexy to have you gently run your fingers through her hair and hold her hair back from her face during a blowjob. But it's NOT sexy to have our hair pulled or our head held/forced in a certain position.
- So often men focus on getting that blowjob and consider it a successful night if they get one. If you're one of those guys that are consumed with BJs, let me clue you in

on something very, very important...women get absolutely NOTHING out of them. You are in no way turning her on during a blowjob. So, BJs cannot be the only form of foreplay you have for the evening. Keep this in mind as you feel yourself getting closer and closer to cumming during that blowjob--you're going to have to take some time after it to get her going too. Even if you've put time into foreplay BEFORE the BJ, you will have to go back to it again afterwards also.

- Is there ever a time where you can get JUST a blowjob without sex? Yes, but let her seduce you with it--in other words you can't demand it and it only.

- What if I don't want her giving me a blowjob? You should maybe explore why you don't want this and then have this discussion with her sometime when you're just lying around together, but not when you're trying to have sex. Giving her some of your reasons why will let her know that it's not anything to do with her, but rather with the act itself and that it wouldn't matter who it was trying to do it.

- If she has a cold sore do not let her go down on you, and the same goes for you going down on her with one.

- The best time to squeeze a BJ in during a sex session is before you put your penis in any other hole.
- It's insulting and rude to expect women to give blowjobs just because they're on their period. It doesn't matter what part of the month it is, it doesn't change the fact that we don't get any sexual stimulation AT ALL from a BJ--so keeping this in mind, be ready to do other things besides a BJ during our period.
- Not all women swallow. It's important to always give her enough warning before you ejaculate so she can decide how she's going to deal with it, and never, ever force it. This is more about being a gentleman than anything else. Women like gentlemen.

That's about it on this subject. If you're wondering if I have a book out on blowjobs, I don't--not yet anyway! Stay tuned.

Let's talk about: Social Media

This is the easiest thing to write about when it comes to advice on how it fits into a new relationship.

Here's the advice in a nutshell: do not put ANYTHING on social media about a new relationship, and then, after the relationship is established, put as little as possible on social media. Social media brings out all the ex's and jealous friends/acquaintances and can cause problems that aren't really there. Keep anything that means a lot to you OFF of all social media platforms.

<u>Let's talk about: What You Tell the Boys</u>

It's best to not tell your boys much about any women that you're dating, but if you want to join in with their rowdy boasting, then do so in generalities. Don't ever give up details about the girl you are currently seeing or any of your ex-girlfriends from the last five years. Why five years? Well, you never know if one of your friends will end up with one of your ex's. If, after five years, no one's hooked up with her then it's probably okay to talk about her since she's more than likely moved on out of your social circle. Nothing like talking in detail about a woman who ends up being married to one of your friends! .
It's also a bad idea to show or share any pictures of your girlfriend with other guys. This can backfire and cause your breakup. It's also considered a crime in many states, so just don't do it. Keep all intimate pictures to yourself.

<u>Let's talk about: Knowing When to Call it Quits</u>

Believe it or not, this is the hardest part to write about...I guess it's because there's never a clear-cut answer.

I can't cover **everything** that might prompt you to think about calling it quits, but here's a few of the more common signs that you should. If you think about someone else more often than you think about your current partner then you should probably be asking yourself why, and then get out. If you dread going home, or going anywhere with your partner, then you should give them up. If you're drinking more than usual just because you're having to spend time with your partner, then you should end it.

Also keep in mind that just because it's a long-term relationship shouldn't be a reason to stick it out if you're unhappy. You may have invested months, or years, into a relationship but that doesn't mean that that relationship is going to for sure be your "end-all". People change. Relationships change. And both sometimes grow at different rates, and in different directions...and that's okay. Letting go means you're trying to embrace something better--something that makes you happier.

It's hard to break up, but that's certainly not a good reason for not doing it if you're unhappy. It's up to you and your partner if you want to try couples counseling or other ways to save your relationship, but generally, it's all boils down to not having a strong emotional connection.

    And THAT's what **good** sex can help make, and preserve, in a relationship--physical and emotional connections that can ultimately lead to a fulfilling life. This is my motivation for putting out this manual...I want you to have the secret to building a strong, intimate, fulfilling relationship that will provide you with the love, passion and acceptance that all of us humans crave.

    I hope this book has answered all of your questions, but if not...check in with your partner, I'm sure they'll be able to help you out! Good luck & have fun!